NOURISH YOUR LIFE

Mastering Appetite

For Abundant Living

KARRY WILSON

ISBN: 9798861334051

Contents

INTRODUCTION

Do you find yourself mindlessly munching to curb cravings or indulging your taste buds, or are you purposefully nurturing your body to seize control of your destiny?

In the digital age, where the world's pace is relentless and well-being is paramount, we embark on a journey through this eBook to unveil the transformative power of mindful eating. It's not just about satisfying your hunger; it's about unlocking the potential within you.

Within these pages, we'll delve into the art of conscious nutrition, exploring how every bite you take can be a stepping stone towards a more fulfilled and vibrant life. Let's embark on this voyage of self-discovery and harness the profound impact of nourishing your body and mind for a future brimming with vitality and success.

CHAPTER 1

The Modern Eating Dilemma

In a world that moves faster than ever before, we've witnessed a radical shift in our eating habits. Gone are the days when a meal was a carefully prepared dish, savored with intention and appreciation.

Today, "I am hungry" often translates to grabbing a quick, processed meal - a burger, hot dog, and a side of fries, perhaps washed down with a sugary cola. "Let's go out and party" now frequently means a night of excessive drinking, interspersed with synthetic-laden fast food. And when someone says, "I am on a diet," it often means reliance on chemically driven appetite suppressants, devoid of essential nutrients.

It's no wonder that our collective health is spiraling downward. Our eating choices are not just individual problems; they are global issues. This situation isn't unique to the U.S.; it plagues most so-called developed nations.

Are we reflecting on this? Regrettably, we often aren't. As you read this guide, there might be a bag of processed snacks nearby. Do you realize that these snacks, laden with some of the most harmful chemicals, could have instead nourished a malnourished child in underdeveloped nations?

However, this isn't just about philanthropy; it's about self-preservation. With alarming health statistics, aren't we inviting doom upon ourselves? It's clear that our eating habits have gone astray, leading to an excess baggage of obesity and its related health issues. It's time to take stock of our choices and their implications for our well-being.

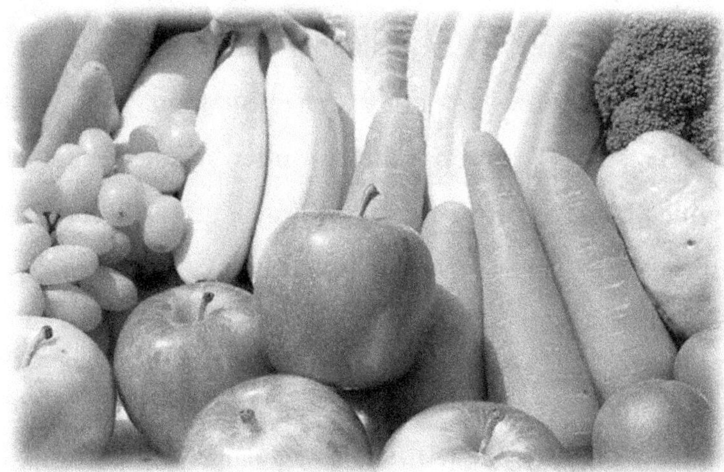

CHAPTER 2

Embracing the Road to Health

Our eating habits have led us down a treacherous path, and it's high time we course-corrected. The key to transformation begins with awareness. We must equip ourselves with the knowledge of what foods truly nurture our bodies and the appropriate portions in which they should be consumed.

Think of it as a journey back to school – not in the traditional sense, but as an opportunity to understand the nutritional needs of our bodies comprehensively. Armed with this knowledge, we can craft a dietary blueprint for ourselves and our families that promotes healthier eating habits. This isn't a sermon; it's a lifeline.

The truth is, we need to cut back on foods that harm us – the excess carbohydrates, fats, and sugars that offer little to no benefit. Instead, we should welcome foods that fortify our health. It might sound preachy, but it's our most potent recourse. Munching on Oreos won't lead to improvement; it's time to break the cycle.

Hope, however, remains within reach. There are countless foods that are equally delicious, yet we remain unaware of them. These undiscovered culinary gems may be unfamiliar or unappetizing to us, but with the right guidance, we can unlock their potential for healthy, delectable meals.

A well-crafted health cookbook, for instance, can introduce us to exciting ways of preparing nutritious dishes. Even with our current dietary staples, we can whip up mouthwatering, health-conscious meals. The possibilities are endless, and we can make substantial modifications to our eating habits while keeping our taste buds delighted.

It's important to acknowledge that the weight loss industry plays a significant role in perpetuating our health crisis. They promote diets like Atkins, Jenny Craig, Zone, and Medifast, and the media often fails to illuminate the simple solutions we can implement independently. Those dramatic before-and-after photos of individuals with miraculous transformations aren't just the result of diets – they are the outcome of taking control of one's life.

So, what do we need to do? It's quite straightforward:

Take charge of what we eat.

Engage in regular physical activity.

Is it too much to ask? Don't we owe it to our bodies, which have faithfully served us all these years? Don't we owe it to ourselves and our families?

Throughout this guide, we'll explore how we can cultivate healthier eating habits and modify our diets to enhance our lives significantly. It's not just a possibility; it's a reality waiting to be embraced.

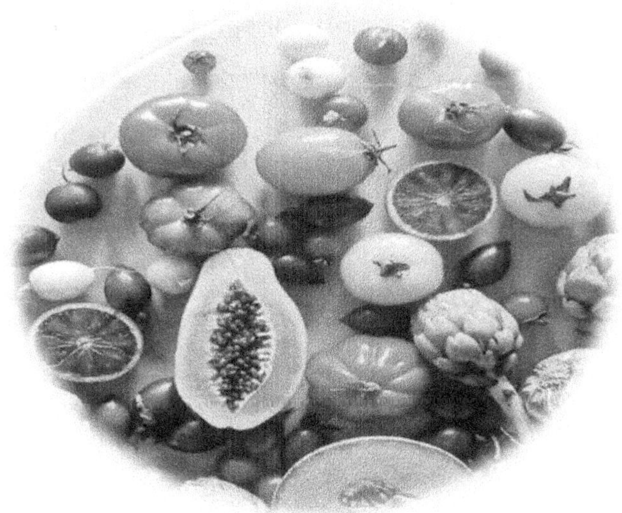

CHAPTER 3

Crafting Your Ideal Diet

Defining an ideal diet is like trying to hit a moving target because it's highly individualized. What constitutes an ideal diet for one person may not hold true for another. Diet perfection is shaped by various factors, including lifestyle, age, gender, physical activity levels, and even geographic location and climate.

One crucial consideration when tailoring a diet is the daily caloric intake, which varies significantly among individuals based on their physical activity. Let's take a closer look at different categories of individuals and their recommended daily calorie consumption to help establish their ideal diets.

Caloric Requirements by Lifestyle and Gender

Men leading a sedentary life: 2,300 calories per day

Men involved in high physical activity: 3,200 calories per day

Women leading a sedentary life: 2,000 calories per day

Women involved in high physical activity: 2,500 calories per day

Pregnant women: 2,500 calories per day

Lactating women: 3,000 calories per day

Infants up to a year-old: 50 calories for each pound of body weight

Children between 1 and 10 years: 1,000 – 2,000 calories per day

Teenage boys: 2,000 – 2,500 calories per day

Teenage girls: 1,500 – 2,000 calories per day

While ideal diets differ from person to person, some universal principles can guide everyone toward healthier eating:

Balanced Carbohydrates: Ensure an adequate but not excessive intake of carbohydrates. Excess carbohydrates can lead to glucose buildup in the body.

Minimize Fried Foods: Limit fried foods to one serving per day, if at all. Excessive consumption of fried foods can have adverse health effects.

Embrace Vibrant Veggies: Incorporate green vegetables into your meals. A general rule of thumb is that colorful foods are often more nutritious, although there are exceptions both ways. Some colorless foods are highly nutritious (think cabbage), while colorful foods may lack essential nutrients.

Choose Lean Meats: Opt for lean meats, and maintain a balanced ratio between non-vegetarian and vegetable components in your meals to ensure a healthier balance.

Mindful Cooking: Cook your food just enough to retain its natural flavors and nutrients. While spices enhance taste, they can also deplete nutritional value, so use them judiciously.

Avoid Synthetics: Eliminate synthetic materials from your diet. Processed foods loaded with artificial additives should be excluded.

Remember that your ideal diet is not a rigid formula but a set of guidelines that should adapt to your unique needs. Crafting a personalized diet that aligns with your lifestyle and nurtures your health is a continuous journey.

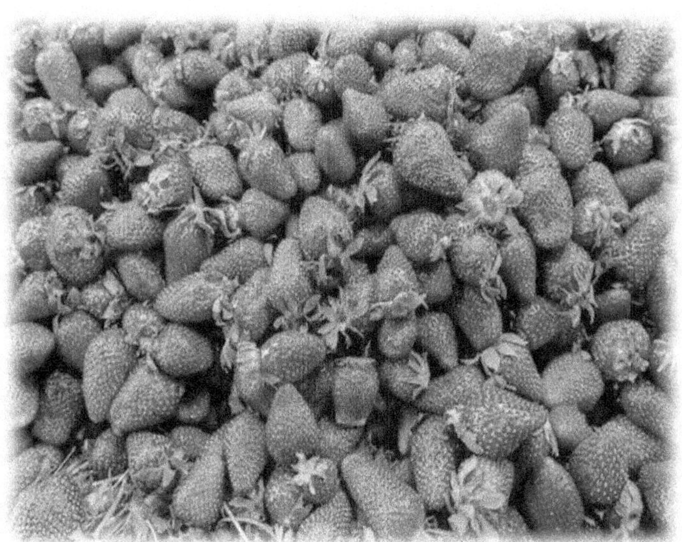

CHAPTER 4

Unlocking the Power of Eating Right

The benefits of eating right extend far beyond just the realm of weight control. Let's delve into this topic and explore the myriad advantages of adopting a healthier diet.

Enhanced Health

While the health benefits of proper nutrition are vast, one of the most significant is the ability to take control of your weight. Eating right ensures that your metabolic functions, including your immune and digestive systems, operate optimally. Moreover, it shields you from a range of chronic diseases, from cardiovascular conditions like atherosclerosis and high blood pressure to diabetes.

Financial Gains

Choosing a healthy diet often translates into significant savings. Your supermarket bills decrease substantially, and you're less likely to accumulate credit card debt due to excessive spending on unhealthy food choices. Furthermore, you'll save a substantial amount on healthcare expenses that might otherwise result from unhealthy eating habits.

Reduced Toxins

Many modern foods contain synthetic chemicals that can be toxic to your body. By embracing a proper diet, you minimize your exposure to these toxins since a fundamental principle of eating right is avoiding synthetic ingredients.

Additionally, when you consume fewer calories and adopt a healthier lifestyle, you may naturally reduce or eliminate vices like smoking and excessive alcohol consumption. Fewer calories can mean fewer cravings for that post-meal cigarette or night out with friends.

Increased Activity

Improved nutrition often leads to increased productivity. When you eat better, you'll likely find that you have more energy and vitality, allowing you to work, exercise, travel, play, and enjoy life to the fullest. This is a far cry from a sedentary lifestyle that results from poor dietary choices, where you might spend most of your day on the couch.

Enhanced Social Life

It's no secret that society often places importance on physical appearance. Excess weight can influence not only your self-esteem but also your social interactions. Obesity can hinder your ability to find a partner and can lead to social stigmatization.

People may perceive individuals who struggle to control their eating habits as lacking self-discipline. However, when you make the choice to eat right, these barriers begin to dissolve, and your social life can flourish.

By embracing the benefits of a healthier diet, you're not only investing in your physical health but also enhancing your financial well-being, reducing exposure to harmful toxins, increasing your activity levels, and enriching your social life. It's a transformative journey that pays dividends in multiple aspects of your life.

CHAPTER 5

The Blueprint for Successful Weight Loss

In your quest to shed those extra pounds through proper nutrition, there are vital components that often take precedence over the food you consume. Let's address these fundamental aspects of weight loss, which, when combined with a balanced diet, will maximize your chances of success.

Motivation: Your North Star

Losing weight effectively begins with motivation. It's the driving force that keeps you committed to your goals.

This objective can vary from person to person, whether it's the desire to enhance your appearance, improve your health, boost physical activity levels, or achieve any other personal aspiration. Once you've identified your goal, focus on it relentlessly. This unwavering dedication helps chart your path to success.

The Power of Support and Encouragement

While some individuals embark on weight loss journeys independently, having a support system can significantly simplify the process.

Family and friends who offer encouragement and positive reinforcement, rather than criticism, play a vital role. Their belief in your journey can be a strong motivator. For some, the desire to be more productive in family life can serve as a compelling reason to shed excess weight.

Participating in a weight loss program with a companion can also be highly effective. A touch of healthy competition can provide that extra push you need to stay on track. The friendly rivalry and shared goals can make the journey both enjoyable and rewarding.

Now, let's address the dietary component.

Resist Fad Diets: Focus on Your Health Plan

Amid the multitude of food fads circulating on the internet, it's crucial to remain grounded in reality. These fad diets are often unnecessary and unsustainable.

Instead, what truly matters is your determination and your ability to make informed food choices.

Develop a comprehensive health plan tailored to your specific needs and adhere to it diligently. Such plans can yield excellent results without the need for fad diets. You have the potential to become your own fitness expert, utilizing your unique goals and requirements as a guide.

In the end, the key to successful weight loss lies not in trendy diets but in your unwavering motivation, a solid support system, and a personalized health plan. These elements, coupled with sensible food choices, will pave the way for a healthier, slimmer you.

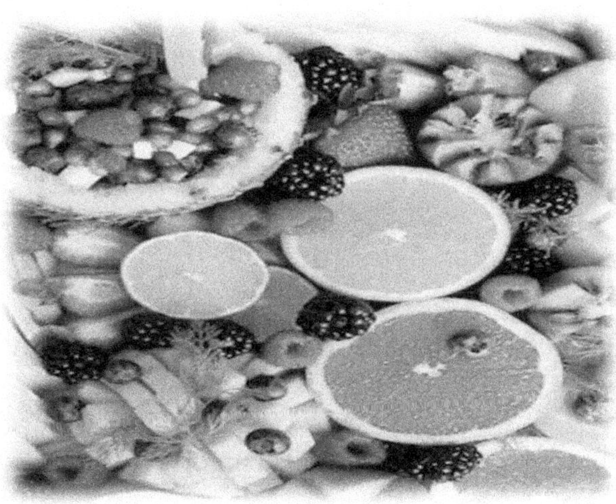

CHAPTER 6

Beyond Diet: The Holistic Approach to Wellbeing

You've undoubtedly heard the refrain that a healthy lifestyle involves more than just proper nutrition. While diet plays a pivotal role, it's merely one piece of the puzzle. Physical activity often springs to mind as a crucial supplement to diet, and rightfully so.

We're well aware of the numerous benefits of regular exercise. However, there are several other facets to consider when enriching your life alongside healthy eating and exercise. Let's explore this holistic approach to wellbeing.

The Power of a Positive Attitude

Optimism and enthusiasm for life can significantly impact your overall wellbeing. A positive attitude serves as a cornerstone of a fulfilling life. It can empower you to excel in various aspects of your existence.

Mindful Stress Management

Stress is an unavoidable part of modern life, but how you manage it can greatly influence your health.

Incorporating stress management techniques such as meditation, deep breathing exercises, or even engaging in hobbies can foster emotional equilibrium.

Adequate Rest and Sleep

Quality sleep is an essential pillar of a healthy lifestyle. It's during slumber that your body regenerates and repairs itself.

Adequate rest and sleep contribute to enhanced cognitive function, emotional stability, and overall vitality.

Stay Hydrated

Proper hydration is often overlooked but is indispensable for bodily functions.

Water facilitates digestion, maintains body temperature, and ensures the optimal performance of vital organs. Incorporate ample water intake into your daily routine.

Cultivate Strong Relationships

Human connection is fundamental to wellbeing. Nurturing meaningful relationships with family, friends, and your community can provide emotional support, reduce stress, and contribute to a sense of belonging.

Continual Learning and Growth

A curious and open mind is an asset. Engage in lifelong learning and personal growth. Expanding your knowledge, whether through reading, taking courses, or pursuing new skills, fosters mental agility and fulfillment.

Practice Gratitude

Taking time to acknowledge and appreciate the positive aspects of your life can enhance your overall happiness. Gratitude promotes emotional wellbeing and can improve your outlook on life.

Regular Health Check-ups

Scheduled health check-ups and screenings are essential to catch potential health issues early. Early detection and intervention can often prevent more severe health complications.

While a balanced diet and exercise are crucial components of a healthy lifestyle, they are part of a more comprehensive picture.

Embrace a holistic approach to wellbeing, considering physical, emotional, and social factors. By doing so, you'll unlock the true potential of a fulfilling and healthy life.

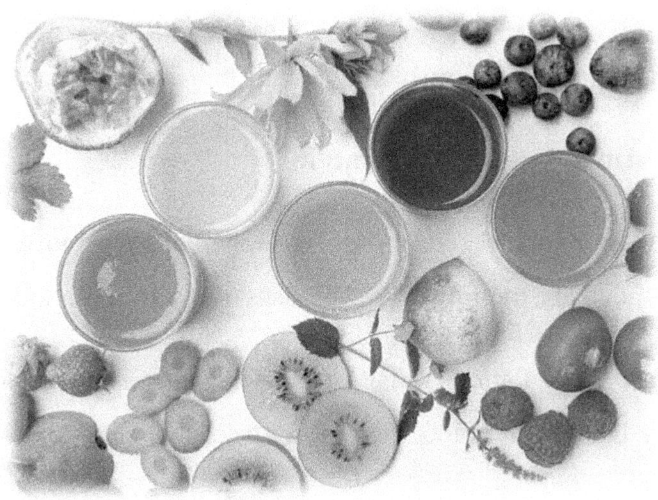

CHAPTER 7

Balancing Healthy Eating with Social Life

Entering a journey of healthy eating often brings unexpected challenges, particularly in the realm of social interactions. Here are some common scenarios and strategies for managing food choices while maintaining relationships with family and friends.

Scenario 1: Family Frustrations

"I started a natural eating program for my kids at home, and now they hate me for it." – A housewife with three kids.

Modern Approach: Transitioning your family to healthier eating habits can indeed be met with resistance.

Instead of sudden, drastic changes, involve them in the process. Consider having "healthy recipe nights" where everyone helps prepare nutritious meals.

Explain the benefits of these changes in a way that's understandable to each family member.

Scenario 2: Relationship Tensions

"Did I do something wrong? My husband thinks I am more obsessive about my waistline than I am about him." – A 20-year old wife.

Modern Approach: Balancing personal health goals and relationships requires open communication. Discuss your intentions and share your desire for a healthier lifestyle with your partner. Involve them in your journey by preparing delicious and nutritious meals together. Highlight how these changes can lead to more energy and vitality, benefiting both of you.

Scenario 3: Social Pressure

"I just missed a party invitation because they thought I wouldn't want the temptation to come my way." – An office-going middle-aged male.

Modern Approach: Maintaining social connections while adhering to your healthy eating plan is crucial. Let your friends and colleagues know that you're committed to a healthier lifestyle, but you also value their company. Suggest alternative social gatherings that align with your dietary goals, like a picnic or outdoor activities.

Resisting the Urge to Preach

People embarking on a healthy eating journey sometimes become zealous advocates, inadvertently alienating friends and family. Instead, share your experiences and insights when they express interest. Be a source of inspiration rather than imposing your choices on others.

Moderation, Not Deprivation

Emphasize that your healthy eating plan allows for occasional indulgences. Communicate that you're flexible and can enjoy a treat now and then. This helps dispel any concerns that you might be too rigid or judgmental.

Your journey to better health is a personal one. While you aspire to influence those around you positively, respect their individual timelines and choices. Ultimately, the goal is to foster a supportive environment where everyone can thrive, both in health and in relationships.

CHAPTER 8

Igniting Your Passion for Healthy Eating

Embarking on a journey toward healthier eating can be daunting. After all, parting ways with familiar indulgences like fried foods and sugary drinks can feel like a seismic shift. But it doesn't have to be a nightmare. In fact, it can be an exciting and empowering adventure. Let's explore new ways to motivate yourself on this path to better health.

Setting a Compelling Goal

Motivation often stems from having a clear and compelling goal. Your goal could be as diverse as wanting to look and feel better, improving your energy levels, rediscovering activities you love, or even proving doubters wrong. The key is to choose a goal that resonates deeply with you.

Modern Tip: Visualize your goal regularly. Create a vision board with images and affirmations related to your aspirations. This visual reminder can be a powerful motivator.

The Power of Resilience

Resilience is your unwavering commitment to stay on track. When you resolve not to give up, you become less likely to deviate from your healthy eating plan. Share this resolution with family, friends, or colleagues, turning them into allies who can gently remind you of your commitment when temptation lurks.

Modern Tip: Use technology to your advantage. There are numerous apps and online communities designed to support your healthy eating journey. Joining a community of like-minded individuals can provide valuable encouragement and accountability.

Fueling Your Passion

Engage in activities that not only excite you but also promote physical activity. Consider taking up hobbies such as swimming or dancing, which become increasingly enjoyable as your body becomes fitter. Not only will these pursuits keep you interested, but they'll also help you shed those extra pounds.

Modern Tip: Explore fitness apps and online classes that cater to your interests. You can learn dance routines or find swimming tutorials online to supplement your physical activity.

The Power of Partnership

Pairing up with someone who shares your health goals can be a game-changer. A partner can provide not only motivation but also friendly competition. As you both progress, you'll celebrate victories together and inspire each other to keep going.

Modern Tip: Consider joining virtual health and fitness challenges with your partner or a group of friends. These challenges often include fun goals and milestones that make the journey more engaging.

Healthy eating is not a confining sentence; it's an opportunity to nurture your well-being and embrace a more vibrant life. By setting a meaningful goal, fostering resilience, pursuing active hobbies, and forging partnerships, you'll find motivation to fuel your journey toward a healthier you.

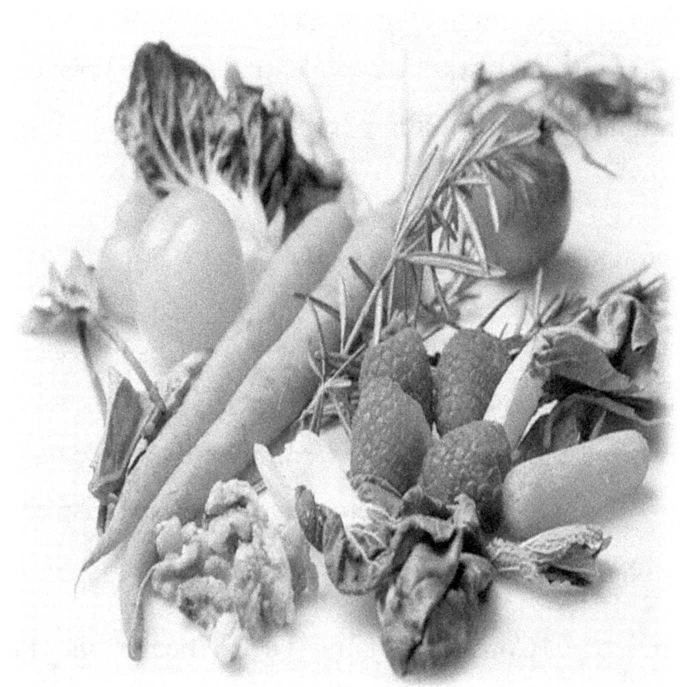

CHAPTER 9

Balancing Your Healthy Eating Journey

While prioritizing healthy eating is essential, it's equally important not to let it consume you.

Obsessing over your diet can lead to stress, nutrient deficiencies, social challenges, and other complications.

Here, we'll explore ways to strike a balance between mindful eating and an obsession-free life.

Understanding the Pitfalls of Obsession

Becoming obsessed with healthy eating can trigger stress responses in your body, releasing cortisol, a hormone that can hinder your metabolism and exacerbate weight issues.

Additionally, excessive restrictions might deprive your body of essential nutrients, potentially leading to dietary deficiencies or even conditions like anorexia.

Maintaining Social Harmony

Your commitment to healthy eating shouldn't become a source of discomfort or inconvenience for those around you.

Consider the impact of your dietary choices on friends and family. Striking a balance between your preferences and their expectations is crucial for maintaining healthy relationships.

Preventing Obsession

To prevent your pursuit of healthy eating from becoming an obsession, consider these strategies:

Occasional Indulgence: Allow yourself occasional treats or cheat days, like a special Sunday dinner with loved ones. This practice not only rewards your dedication but also reinforces a positive relationship with food.

Stress Management: Implement stress-reduction techniques to avoid excessive worry about your diet. Breathing exercises, mindfulness meditation, and yoga are effective ways to maintain mental balance.

Seek Professional Guidance: If you're concerned that your focus on healthy eating is becoming an obsession, consider consulting a registered dietitian or therapist. They can provide valuable insights and strategies to maintain a healthy relationship with food.

Variety in Your Diet: Embrace a diverse range of foods that align with your health goals. Experiment with new recipes and cuisines to keep your meals exciting and satisfying.

Remember, the ultimate goal of eating right is not just physical well-being but also a healthier and happier life. By finding a balance between your dietary choices and the overall quality of your life, you can enjoy the benefits of healthy eating without it becoming an unhealthy obsession.

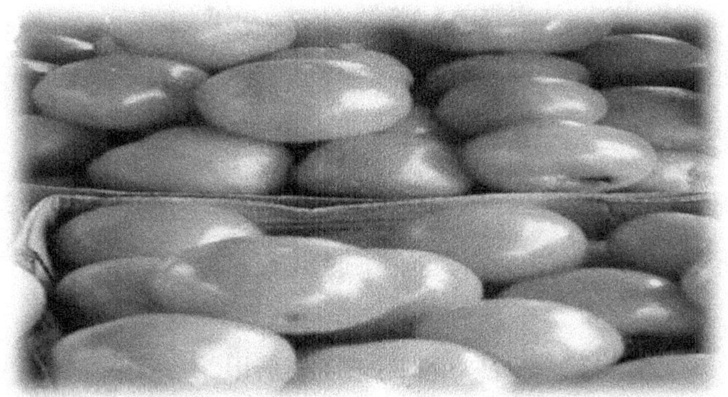

CHAPTER 10

Transforming Your Life Through Mindful Eating

When you embark on a journey of mindful eating, you'll soon discover that it's not just your diet that changes; your entire life begins to transform. Here, we explore how the power of eating right can enable you to seize control of your life and why maintaining your commitment is essential.

Sustaining Your Drive

You might have initiated your "eat right" journey to shed a few extra pounds, but as you progress, you'll realize it's about more than just weight loss. It's a lifestyle shift that empowers you to make healthier choices across the board. It's vital to maintain this momentum. Here's why:

Imagine you've successfully maintained a healthy eating regimen for a few months, and you've seen positive changes in your body. It might be tempting to loosen the reins and indulge in old habits. However, it's crucial to recognize that the true impact of this lifestyle change unfolds over time.

The Two-Month Mark

Studies suggest that if you commit to a healthy eating program for roughly two months, it's more likely to become a lifelong habit. This relatively short duration of dedication can lead to lifelong rewards. The benefits you experience during these two months will motivate you to stay on track.

Seeking Inspiration

To keep your motivation high, delve into resources that inspire you. Read books, watch videos, scour the internet for stories of individuals who have transformed their lives through mindful eating. These real-life examples can provide the motivation you need to continue on your path.

Unlocking a Better Life

By consistently eating right, you're not only achieving physical improvements but also enhancing your overall quality of life. Whether you're seeking to boost your physical performance, increase your stamina, or shed unwanted weight, mindful eating is the key.

However, the most significant transformation occurs in your relationships. You'll find that you have more meaningful and quality time to spend with your loved ones. Nurturing these connections is the true essence of managing your life.

In summary, mindful eating isn't just about food; it's a catalyst for positive change in every aspect of your life. Stay committed for those crucial two months, and you'll unlock the door to a healthier, happier, and more fulfilling life.

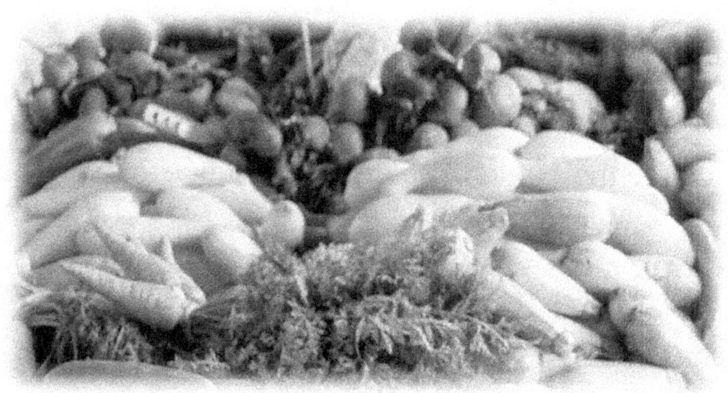

Conclusion

Taking control of your life is a journey you embark on willingly, and one of the most effective paths to empowerment is mindful eating. You've discovered what this means for you, and now it's time to take the next step.

Crafting Your Healthy Eating Journey

Today, you have the knowledge and insight to design a healthy eating plan that suits your unique needs and goals. It's not just about the food you consume; it's about nourishing your body, mind, and spirit with intention and awareness.

Embrace the Transformation

As you venture into this transformative journey, remember that you are not alone. Countless individuals worldwide are on similar paths, seeking to enrich their lives through mindful choices. Your journey starts with a single step towards a healthier, happier, and more fulfilling life.

Your path to a better life begins now. Embrace it with enthusiasm and determination, knowing that the power to manage your life rests in your hands. May your pursuit of mindful eating bring you lasting wellness, strength, and a profound connection to the incredible journey of life itself. The very best of success to you on this empowering adventure!